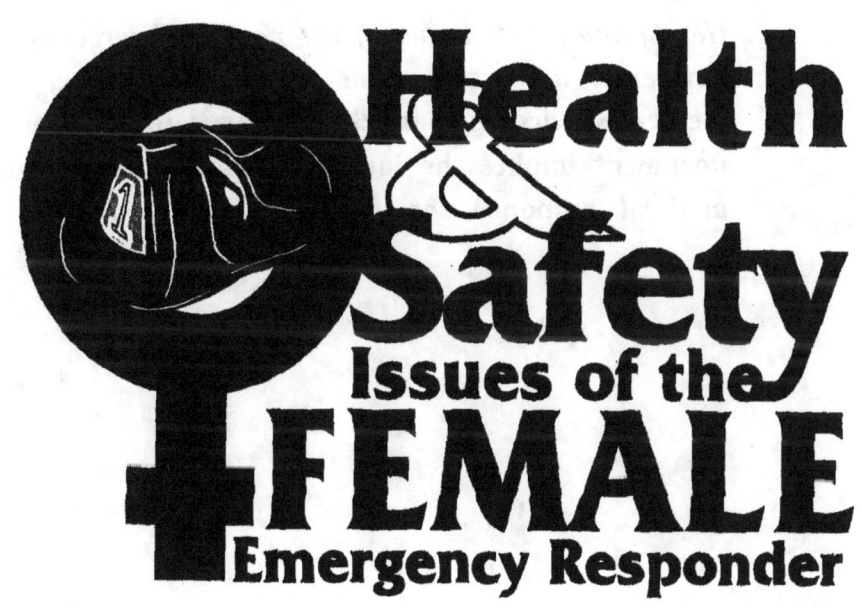

Federal Emergency Management Agency / United States Fire Administration

Health and Safety Issues of the Female Emergency Responder was developed in consideration of all fire, rescue, and emergency medical services personnel. Reference to the fire service in this document implies the inclusion of fire, rescue, and emergency medical response services.

This publication was prepared for the Federal Emergency Management Agency's U.S. Fire Administration under contract No. EMW-94-C-4519. Any opinions, findings, conclusions, or recommendations expressed in this publication do not necessarily reflect the views of the Federal Emergency Management Agency or the United States Fire Administration.

Preface

The U.S. Fire Administration (USFA) publication, *A Handbook on Women in Firefighting-The Changing Face of the Fire Service,* published in 1993, provided basic information concerning the status of women in the profession. The handbook updated and documented information and resources gathered from the USFA's first meeting in 1979 on "Women in the Fire Service," through the monumental increases of women in the fire, rescue; and emergency medical services in the 1980s and early 1990s. The publication reflected more than a decade of experience and progress.

As more and more women enter the fire service, health and safety issues of women gain a greater audience. The knowledge base broadens as the number of women moving through the ranks of the fire service increases, providing more accurate information and a means to assess occupational health and safety risks.

It is apparent now, as we approach the second half of the '9Os, that more explicit information on issues of special concern to women in the fire service is needed. To address this concern, the USFA convened the symposium on "Health and Safety Issues of the Female Emergency Responder," in Rosslyn, Virginia, in October 1994. Twenty-seven participants representing a wide range of interest and involvement in fire and emergency response services were brought together to share their expertise and experiences in specific health and safety issues. The participants were charged with the task of narrowing the focus of health and safety concerns and developing strategies to address the issues of women in emergency response services today. They provided a "snap shot" of the situation for women in the response services and identified the critical issues to address in the immediate future.

We are grateful to the symposium participants for their efforts. The report that follows is a result of their deliberations and experience. We are hopeful their recommendations will provide guidance in meeting the health and safety concerns of female first responders as we move toward the next decade.

Table of Contents

Issue Identification Process

Some issues emerging from the inclusion of women in career-level fire suppression have been dealt with extensively, while others remain to be addressed. In 1979, USFA convened a "Women in the Fire Service" seminar. The resulting report, The *Role of Women in the Fire Service,* summarized the issues discussed at the seminar and presented the participants' recommendations and their personal insights. Based on participants' recommendations, USFA in 1980 developed two manuals-a resource directory for recruiting, testing, and training women firefighters, and the *Personnel Management Handbook: Managing the Entry of Women and Minorities.* These publications focused on the legal and management issues relating to recruitment and training of women. In 1993, *A Handbook on Women in Firefighting: The Changing Face of the Fire Service* was published. It deals with issues of a gender-integrated workforce resulting from the increasing numbers of women entering and moving through the ranks of the fire service. The principle issues addressed in the handbook are recruitment, entry-level physical testing, firefighter training, policy development, sexual harassment, cultural diversity training, ongoing support for minorities and women on the job, and protective clothing fit and safety. Since the publication of the 1993 handbook, interest in the specific health and safety issues of female emergency responders has increased. Consequently, in October 1994, USFA convened a symposium to identify these issues and recommend actions to be taken at the federal, state, and local levels.

Several methods were used to ensure that up-to-date topics were brought to the symposium participants for consideration. An extensive literature search was undertaken to provide a basic understanding of issues that are currently being reported. Individuals who were working as first responders, studying issues related to first responders, and working in related fields were identified. Representatives of emergency response organizations were contacted for their recommendations of persons interested in health and safety concerns of female first responders. The individuals named were contacted to determine their willingness to identify significant issues and/or their interest in and availability to participate in the proposed symposium.

1

The potential attendees and others with experience and expertise in the topic areas were asked individually to rank the concerns catalogued in the literature search and suggest other issues of concern. The responses to this query were used to structure the symposium and to develop the working groups.

Prior to the conference, three issues were identified as paramount to women in the fire service: (1) procedures, protocols, and equipment; (2) organizational health and mental health; and (3) reproductive and toxicological concerns. Background materials on these topics and a copy of *A Handbook on Women in Firefighting: The Changing Face of the Fire Service* were sent to the prospective attendees. The symposium comprised a mixture of plenary and focus work-group sessions, with experts speaking on health and safety issues of female firefighters. Each participant was assigned to one of the three focus groups and remained with the group for all small-group work sessions. Each focus group was asked to develop strategies and recommendations in three areas:

- Data Development and Dissemination
- Training (at all levels)
- Equipment Engineering

In their assigned areas, the work groups identified problems, suggested solutions, and set priorities for their recommendations to federal, state, and local jurisdictions. At the end of each session, the focus groups reported their findings in a plenary session where discussions with other symposium participants often led to refinement, additions, or modifications.

The balance of this report presents the recommendations for action made by the Task Force in each of the three areas.

Recommendations

The symposium concluded each day with the focus groups presenting the issues they identified as priorities to be addressed. The most mentioned issues from all groups are arranged in the three categories: data development and dissemination, training at all levels, and equipment engineering. The recommendations of the symposium and a brief discussion of each follow.

Data Development and Dissemination

Recommendation

USFA initiate the development of an improved data reporting system in cooperation with the National Institute for Occupational Safety and Health (NIOSH) and/or other institutions that function comparable worker pools.

The database must include gender-specific data; exposure, incident, injury, and illness reporting that provides information on the specific situation and mechanism, medical history, and regular follow-up; and a provision for confidentiality.

Currently firefighter death and injury data are collected by the USFA through the National Fire, Data Center (NFDC), which has established the National Fire Incident Reporting System (NFIRS) to help state and local governments develop fire reporting and analysis capability for their own use and to obtain data that can be used to more accurately assess and subsequently combat the fire problem at a national level. Although there has been a serious effort to collect valid information on firefighter concerns to assist in reducing occupationally related death and injury in the fire service, gender-specific information, generally, is not available. Reporting systems rely on local departments to categorize and report incidents; however, standardization is imperfect. In spite of efforts to bring together these diverse data systems, there are still major discrepancies in reported results, and groups expend much effort and energy that could be better used. Little, if any, gender-specific information is collected on a national basis. If these data were available, some perceived problems could be validated and addressed or eliminated. To accomplish this, a uniform system should be developed to collect this data. Expanding the database to include gender-specific information might provide the opportunity to improve coordination and quality of the entire database. Working with organizations both inside and outside the fire community could provide an objective approach to solving this problem.

Recommendation

A national organization coordinate a process of gathering information to define the range of requirements for all positions in response services.

This information would include the specific job requirements of each position. The data should be refined to provide a checklist for each position or category that could be used as is" or adapted to meet local needs. Such basic guidelines would ensure that hiring practices are based on actual job requirements rather than gender bias.

Inconsistency in hiring procedures was identified as a major problem by the focus groups. Although tasks across the fire service are comparable, qualification standards, applications, and position descriptions are local issues and vary widely throughout the service. Maintaining local control is crucial; however, a standardized list of position/task requirements (knowledge, skills, and abilities) would provide a starting point for local departments in developing position descriptions that fit their needs and provide the basis of comparability throughout the fire service. A major benefit of the checklist would be in separating "real requirements" from "what's been done." Additionally, it could help to record specific career track(s) that could offer comparability nationwide.

Recommendation

USFA develop a national clearinghouse to gather and disseminate information on successful or innovative programs.

Issues of particular interest to women in the fire service are hiring, child care, and structured mentoring programs. The clearinghouse would gather and validate information about programs across the country, so that each organization or locality would not have to invent its own. Sharing program information could lead to a more uniform

4

and successful approach for communities in similar circumstances and would avoid many false starts caused by local jurisdictions feeling their way toward solutions of common problems.

Since local emergency response services have limited resources, it is essential to maximize the benefit of their use. Many departments are facing the health and safety issues identified by the symposium. Attempts to address them locally have met with varying success. Results of these efforts are circulated informally by word-of-mouth and serendipitously in publications. There is neither a standard process of evaluating these efforts nor an explicit mechanism for sharing information on their outcome. The task force stressed the need for a system to validate successes, share information, and help interested states or local jurisdictions identify applicable programs in similar communities that could be adapted or adopted. The group further recommended that a peer assistance component be organized that would bring together people from similar jurisdictions with similar problems to share program information and develop solutions. This would strengthen the information exchange system. Using the peer model, individuals who have initiated successful programs addressing specific problems might coach or consult with their counterparts in communities facing similar problems and help build on each department's strengths and minimize the false starts that occur as each department feels its way along.

Recommendation

National and state organizations initiate a serious effort to channel pertinent information to the end user.

Rather than depending on traditional hierarchical distribution channels, efforts must be made to circulate relevant information through the local organization so it timely reaches the end user(s). Information often is sent to the chief or executive of a fire response company, and it may be months before it is filtered down to the line staff who need to implement any changes. The task force noted that the information may never reach the people who need it most.

Training

The second major grouping of recommendations addressed training issues. The recommendations range from general consciousness raising for individuals working in the emergency response services to physician training on the demands of first response work to better meet the health care needs of the first responders who are their patients.

5

Training is needed to move departments toward a more realistic approach to the actual job requirements of the fire service.

Fire and response service leaders must realize that their attitudes toward and interactions with women in their departments set a pattern of behavior to be followed by the rest of the force. As the composition and role of the fire service evolves from an all-male service to one including women at all levels, its leaders must change their views and attitudes to a gender-integrated workforce. Research conducted for the symposium and the reports of symposium participants indicate that some progress has been made; however, much of the fire service needs to improve in this area.

NFA provides training for current and future leaders of the fire service and allied professions and affords the opportunity to inform them of the health and safety concerns discussed at this symposium, familiarize them with sources of problems, and present them with possible solutions. The physical issues raised by gender diversity in the response services are considered to be the primary issues and differences in much the same way that the health professions address disease vectors. They are clear and measurable and relatively concrete.

It is important for the fire service to recognize that women and men often approach tasks differently. This can be as straightforward as using upper body strength to lift versus using one's legs, or it can be as complex as the development of a working structure. A major difference in the working structure of women and men lies in the development of networks versus hierarchies. This is a particularly important difference in the fire service, which is structured hierarchically.

> working life has an impact on the mental and physical
> health of women comparable to that found in men. In
> both cases the effect is strong....The findings also

6

show that the sources of stress in women's lives are more diverse and diffuse than those experienced by men. These differences in the basic daily experience of men and women suggest the need for more research into life course and experiences differentiated by sex. (Poitrast and Zenz 1994)

Recommendation

A study be undertaken to identify the variety of ways tasks can be accomplished successfully and encourage states and local training institutes to incorporate task attainment options in safety training for all fire service personnel.

According to task force participants and current literature, training today is based on standardized practices that do not allow variation.

training techniques are designed to instruct male firefighters who have a higher center of gravity and more upper body strength than women. By disregarding methods that consider these differences, fire departments consequently overlook techniques that could benefit men too. Progressive training officers are realizing that some of the tactics women use to manipulate heavy equipment or gain entry into buildings are more efficient in general. (Hirschman 1993)

A specific example of an inflexible operating procedure is seen in the reaction to women using two hands and a foot for leverage when starting a chain saw. According to Hirschman, some male officers prohibit the adaptation, saying, "Do it my way or don't do it at all."

It's odd how they'll refuse to let a woman perform a task differently from a man but will allow a left-handed male firefighter to accommodate his unique needs even if that involves a slight change in procedure. (Hirschman 1993)

In any case, the inflexibility of training and protocols is an impediment to the full acceptance of the benefits of gender diversity in the response services.

In physical strength, aerobic capacity, and tolerance to hot environments, there is a wide range of capabilities in men and women, and there is much overlap. Thus, the between-individual variations are more important

7

than the between-sex differences. (Poitrast and Zenz 1994)

Recommendation

USFA work with the medical community to develop a program designed to acquaint health care professionals with the work of first responders and the demands of the profession.

Primary care physicians would be targeted so they would be better able to treat sick or injured response personnel appropriately. The current national trend is to reduce medical costs by encouraging speedy return to work after an illness or injury. As a result, individuals are released by their personal physicians to return to work sooner than they actually are able to resume their duties. Working with medical and professional associations to inform practitioners of the specific demands of response personnel could improve this situation.

Although the number of working women continues to increase dramatically, studies of women in the workforce are relatively few, and studies of women in the response services professions are rare. Medical decisions are made and treatments administered in the absence of relevant data and ahead of available science. (Poitrast and Zenz 1994) Providing physicians with up-to-date and good information about the demands of response services could help to close this gap.

Equipment

The third major category of recommendations made by the symposium relates to equipment and facilities.

Recommendation

USFA work with NIOSH, the National Fire Protection Association (NFPA), and national associations of fire and rescue personnel to develop a system for providing manufacturers of clothing and equipment with information on the diverse needs of the response community and work to incorporate these considerations into protective gear products.

One of the ongoing problems for women in nontraditional careers is the lack of availability of appropriately sized clothing and equipment. In 1990, Women in the Fire Service (WFS) conducted a national survey of women firefighters to which more than 400 women responded. "Eighty percent of the women reported that they had experienced fit problems with protective gear or uniforms at some time during their firefighting service; 45% of the career firefighters.. .indicated that they still had problems with one or more items of ill-fitting gear. . . ." (FEMA/USFA 1993) These problems range from the simple discomfort of trousers that are simply "sized down" men's patterns to boots, gloves, and facemasks that are too large to function effectively. Women have reported their oversized gloves make it impossible to hold anything. Although some progress has been made, protective clothing fit-and-safety problems continue, apparently because the purchasing pool is too small and diverse, and major equipment manufacturers are reluctant to focus on them. Bringing together all interested parties to discuss appropriately sized clothing and equipment may improve the situation for females in the firefighting services.

Recommendation

Convene a design task force to work toward national application of health and safety information in the design of equipment and facilities.

The human factors engineering discipline has developed a body of information that could be used as a starting point. Today, women increasingly are pursuing careers in nontraditional occupations, including the military services and the astronaut corps. Both NASA and the military services have conducted human engineering studies in almost all aspects of the newly integrated jobs. The NASA studies included data on the range, size, strength, and reach of potential human crews. The military services studied the capabilities of potential equipment operators and adjustments that would make equipment accessible to all personnel. Applying the information gathered in these studies to the needs of response services would provide a starting point for addressing equipment problems for fire service personnel.

Recommendation

USFA ensure that the full diversity of the fire service is represented in groups that develop equipment and facility designs.

Including members who are representative of the diversity of the service on design task forces might eliminate the potential of working in good faith on a design but missing the need for change or modification because it is not understood. In response services, as in other organizations, it is customary to draw upon experience in developing policies and procedures. Equipment manufacturers and facility designers also rely on the information provided by senior representatives of the service as products are developed. Since the service has been male dominated for so many years, representation on committees, panels, and boards that develop policies and materials is also male dominated. In addition, participation in these bodies often is at the individuals' expense. Because women in the service are, for the most part, at an earlier stage of career development, they may not have the time or financial means to take part in these groups. Although participation or membership may be open and even encouraged, circumstances serve to keep the policy cycle closed. Full representation is imperative if the specific concerns of the diverse membership of the service are to be equitably addressed. However well meaning the majority individual, he cannot see issues from the minority perspective; thus, concerns of the diverse workforce are not adequately addressed. Symposium participants recognize that full participation as these issues are confronted is critical, and achieving full representation may require some support, at least initially.

Mental Health

Recommendation

Members of the fire service and local, state, and national organizations should work to ensure the acceptance of mental health claims by insurance companies as equal to physical injury claims.

The group recognized that both mental health and stress are major issues in first response. Twelve psychic stress factors that may be present in the workplace have been identified (Elo 1994):

> Responsibility for safety
> Responsibility for other people
> Responsibility for material values (equipment and materials)
> Solitary work
> Burdensome contacts
> Repetitiveness
> Forced pace
> Structural restraints (following specific procedures)

Demands for attentiveness combined with few stimuli
Demands for precise discrimination
Haste
Demands for complex decision making

It is apparent that a large percentage of these stress factors are present in emergency response work. Recent research on sleep deficit, post-traumatic stress, and burnout among paramedics indicates that stress is an ever present factor in emergency response services. Given the high level of stress factors and the close linkage between stress, mental and physical health, and job performance, it would be beneficial to support mental health care in the same way that physical wellness care is supported.

Other Recommendations

The symposium proposed additional recommendations that did not fit into the specific categories assigned to the focus groups. Topics included full participation, research, evaluation and accreditation, and standards.

Full Participation

Recommendation

Include women as full participants in all phases of policy development, to include local committees, state boards, national forums, and NFPA policy committees.

A support system to provide funding to launch "full participation" of women at all levels may be required.

Research

Recommendation

Undertake research on the effects of heat, cold, noise, and radiation on female first responders and on long-term injury and illness related to wildland incidents.

Several current studies show that handling and processing of certain materials are gender specific.

11

Evaluation and Accreditation

Recommendation

Program standards that are developed to promote diversity and acceptance should be applied in an accreditation process prior to disseminating and replicating the programs nationwide.

Accreditation programs should reflect training and ongoing recruitment, and accreditation and standards bodies must reflect women's issues in published standards and standard setting meetings.

Standards

Recommendation

Support the adoption of NFPA 1500, as a way to promote basic health and safety standards expeditiously.

Recommendation

Develop non-gender-biased performance standards that promote diversity and acceptance and have women represented in all areas of decision making.

Perspective

Women first entered the career firefighting service only two decades ago. Although women have served in emergency medical and volunteer fire protection roles for centuries, the career fire service was an all-male workforce. In 1979, the USFA convened a seminar, *Women in the Fire Service,* in College Park, Maryland. The fire service leaders who participated in this seminar discussed issues related to the phenomenon of women employed as firefighters. At that time, there were only a few hundred female firefighters nationwide. The proceedings of that seminar were published in *The Role of Women in the Fire Service.* The publication summarized the issues discussed at the seminar, presented the recommendations of the participants, and provided a list of current initiatives and resources.

In 1980, two additional documents were published. The first was a resource directory of fire departments that had experience in employing, recruiting, and training women firefighters. The second, a handbook entitled *Personnel Management Handbook: Managing the Entry of Women and Minorities,* dealt with the legal and management issues related to opening the fire service to women.

When women first joined the Chicago Fire Department in 1987, the situation was described as:

> firehouses were where *men* lived. And *men* only. Sure they had wives, children, and owned a home. And on days off, they mowed lawn, shoveled the walks, tiled the downstairs bathroom, and put in a patio. But every third day, for 24 hours straight, they lived in the firehouse, and that was their home too. It was where they swaggered around with the ease of men among men.

> They could be tough on each other, but there was an understanding. They could be crude, but they were close. If they were busy in a firehouse, they fought fires together and grew even closer-counting on each other day after day, watching each other's backs and saving each other's hides. If they were in a quiet firehouse, they still had a good time together.

> But no matter the firehouse, you had to fit in to survive. There were the written rules of "the department" and the unwritten rules

of the firehouse. But they were men's rules. And the men all were brothers. (Kegan 1991)

Women were not welcomed into this male bastion, or in many others across the country; they earned their way in and the respect of their colleagues by demonstrating they wanted to work and to learn. This happened in many ways, but for the most part, the women who joined the Chicago Fire Department were accepted.

Twelve years later, the number of women working in the fire service had increased substantially. Women had been promoted through the ranks to district and battalion chief positions, and some forces were as much as 10 percent women. The USFA reviewed the changes that had occurred in the fire service and determined that the information in the previous three handbooks should be updated. Thus, *A Handbook on Women in Firefighting: The Changing Face of the Fire Service,* was published in January 1993. It focused on issues of recruitment; entry-level physical testing; reproductive and child-care policy development; sexual harassment; and protective clothing fit and safety; among others. The purpose was to provide a resource useful to all fire service personnel, whatever their activities in integrating women into the service. Olin Greene, then USFA Administrator, states in the preface that "USFA is committed to promoting an environment where women and men can work harmoniously and productively together to protect our communities. " (FEMA/USFA 1993) The quest for that diverse and harmonious environment continues today. Although there are now over three thousand women in the career fire service, there are many departments and companies where "the brand new experience of hiring a woman into an all male world" is repeated regularly, even today.

With the growing number of women in the fire service comes a greatly increased interest in health and safety issues specific to women. Based on the experiences of women who are moving through the ranks, information is available that allows a better assessment of the health and safety risks facing women in the fire service. Among the concerns identified are:

- Stress management
- Size and fit of protective clothing
- Reproductive health

In addition to these concerns, the increasing number of emergency responses to incidents involving hazardous radioactive, chemical, or biological materials makes it essential that we identify and address risks for the well-being of all in the service. The challenge to the fire and response services and the environment in which they operate ensures the health and safety of personnel by employing the most effective administrative and engineering controls available to resolving these issues.

As USFA looked at the experiences of departments across the nation, they recognized that attempts had been made to address the issues raised by the new diverse face of the response services. More specific information was needed in order to focus efforts and ensure that priority issues were on its agenda. Thus, in October 1994, USFA convened the Task Force Symposium on "Health and Safety Needs of Female Firefighters and First Responders," to assess the occupational health and safety issues of concern to women and to recommend strategies to address the identified needs.

Issue Identification

To ensure that the symposium addressed health and safety issues of most concern to female first responders, questionnaires were sent to 100 individuals, female first responders, fire chiefs, fire and rescue personnel, and others interested in fire and emergency response services. They were asked to rank the importance of twelve health and safety concerns of female first responders.

Of the twenty-seven responses received, fifteen were from women (55% of total respondents), including eleven female first responders. The rankings of the female first responders were used to identify the health and safety issues to be addressed at the symposium and to structure the work of the focus groups. They are presented below in order of ranking, as determined by those respondents. What is most significant is the ranking of "increased risk of heart attack, " considered by all groups of respondents to be of least concern. In reality, heart attack is the number one killer of firefighters.

1. Stress related to 'fitting in' in a nontraditional occupation is a health problem for women first responders.

2. Personal protective equipment (PPE) not designed to fit properly is a health and safety concern.

   Exposure to toxic substances and their possible effect on reproductive health is a concern to women first responders.

3. Stress related to tasks required on the job is a concern for women first responders,

   Engineering design of equipment required for the job is appropriate for women first responders.

   Accepted protocols for accomplishing tasks are appropriate for you.

4. Exposure to blood borne pathogens is a primary concern for women first responders.

5. On the job injuries, such as strains and pulls, are a problem for women first responders.

6. Cancer caused by exposure to the products of combustion is a health concern for women in the fire service.

7. Training provides sufficient safety information in areas of specific concern to women first responders.

8. Increased risk of heart attack in comparison to the general population is a health concern for women first responders.

Comments

Respondents were asked to note any issue that was not addressed in the questionnaire but which they considered important for the health and safety of women first responders. The responses are listed below:

<u>**Female First Responders**</u>
Adverse effects of 800 MHz radio systems (NYC EMTs have researched this concern)
Requirements to maintain male norm body-fat percentage
Work schedules-shifts and family responsibilities
Furnishing firefighters with better ways to find fire and monitor heat levels
Entry-level physical testing
Stress of annual physical performance tests
Fit of equipment for firefighters of smaller stature
Fitting (acceptance) into the firehouse
Sexual harassment

<u>**Other Women**</u>
High energy expenditure required by firefighting and firefighting gear which can raise the core body temperature and affect reproductive health of mother and fetus.
Very high levels of energy and physical strength required for tasks that could be automated or designed to be less strenuous.
Fitness programs for women
Obtaining health care coverage

<u>**Men**</u>
Validity of physical performance testing and standards
Maintenance of adequate strength to provide a margin of safety and perform job functions
Weight of PPE
Sexual harassment and pressure
Chemicals in breast milk
Effects of excessive noise exposure
Training
Recruitment, selection, and education, whether high school or junior college
Approach to job aimed at "guarantee" of success, which often leads to doing more than required by the job
Political and societal issues equal to health and safety issues
Exposure to diesel exhaust in station

Appendix

Remarks

Agenda

Speakers and
Participants

Suggested Reading

A QUALITATIVE INVESTIGATION OF TRADESWOMEN'S HEALTH AND SAFETY CONCERNS

Linda M. Goldenhar, Ph.D.
National Institute for Occupational Safety and Health
Industrywide Studies Branch

The National Institute for Occupational Safety and Health (NIOSH) is the occupational research branch of the Centers for Disease Control (CDC). It was established to carry out and publish industrywide studies of the effect of chronic or low level exposures to industrial material, processes, and stresses and the potential for illness disease or loss of functional capacity in the population of aging adults.

I am a behavioral scientist and work with social psychological principals, applying them to the area of occupational health and safety. I am particularly interested in the behavioral aspects of occupational health and safety, such as the use of safety equipment and stress on the job as well as in women's issues. Women's health is something that NIOSH is just getting started in and we need to focus more on that.

What we are going to talk about today is my area of specific interest, which is related to women in the construction industry. It is tangentially related to the subject of this meeting because the women in construction have many of the same concerns and issues as women in response services. I hope that you can take what I present, place it in the paradigm of firefighters, and gain from it. Today's talk is about our efforts to identify some of the issues facing women in the industry today.

In 1991 the construction industry employed approximately 600,000 women. Research has shown that for many reasons women are choosing nontraditional careers, probably including fire fighting and emergency response, and will continue to pursue employment in these industries. This strengthens the need to identify and address the health and safety concerns of these women.

The findings I will report on today are part of a research agenda aimed at addressing some of the specific gaps in knowledge that will help enhance the health and safety of women and for that matter men choosing these fields.

The first phase of the study was to use qualitative research methods to obtain attitudinal data for women working in the construction industry. The next phase will be to use these data to develop a survey instrument to assess the psychosocial predictors of health and safety behaviors or the reasons why people do or do not behave in a certain way. The final goal will be to develop and evaluate specific health and safety interventions or solutions based on all of the collected data.

In the first phase, we used focus groups, in-depth interviews, and open-ended surveys. The qualitative measures that were used permit the researcher to elicit information about perceptions, attitudes, and beliefs as seen by the respondents rather than predetermining them. The study used attitudes, and beliefs as seen by the respondents rather than predetermining them. The study used a purposeful sample to collect data from information-rich cases to get a better picture of their health and safety concerns. The sample included twenty-five focus group participants who were already involved in trades groups around the country, five in-depth interviews, and twenty-five open-ended surveys.

The two questions I will discuss today are:

- What, in your opinion, are the two or three most important factors on a construction site that affect health and safety?

- Are there any special health and safety issues on the job faced by women?

Five comprehensive health and safety categories were identified: exposure issues, injuries, education and training, awareness of surroundings, and issues related to being a woman on the job.

Exposure issues are clearly the most important to these women. It is possible that exposure issues are so important because individuals have the least control over areas of exposure at work. In terms of risk perception, people often feel at greatest risk when they have little control. For example, although smoking is clearly a risk, people are more concerned about other issues because they feel they can control their own smoking behavior. As you can imagine, many of the same exposure issues like radiation, workplace noise, lead, and asbestos relate to first responders as well. One of the women said, "My concern is the contractors, what products they are using. Do they have their safety datasheets on hand? Are they actually using proper ventilation procedures? Are they being aware of.. .cigarettes and open flames, where they can create some kind of reaction?" This clearly shows lack of control and a concern about whether other people paying attention to what is appropriate and what is going on.

In terms of injuries, the concern was lifting and bending. One respondent said, ". . . how to lift and how to bend.. .I didn't learn this until I ended up in physical therapy. I think that it's something that we really need to look at, especially for individuals going into nontraditional work, is the way you lift and bend and move. " This is a place where interventions can happen in terms of training and the possibilities are exciting.

Falling and eye injuries and cuts on fingers and hands were mentioned by a number of women. The workers said that to avoid these risks it is important not to become too complacent. It is important to learn how to use tools properly and to always remember that they can hurt or kill you. One woman said ". , . what will hurt someone every time is complacency. We had an electrician get shocked....That's simple complacency. . . you get used to it, you do it every day and you take it for granted." That problem certainly would apply in the fire and rescue area as well. I asked the women what they thought would happen if the industry were female dominated. Would there be the same problems? At first they said of course it would be better, but on reflection they recognized that eventually the women too would get very familiar with the tools and the work and the same problems of complacency would arise.

The third area of concern to these women was education and training, or the lack thereof. Many women entering the construction trade are learning a whole new set of mechanical, technical, and physical skills that men may have picked up informally while they were growing up. Although pre-apprenticeship programs are now available, recruiting efforts and funding for these programs is minimal. In preparing for this meeting, I read *A Handbook on Women in Firefighting* where one woman firefighter described her experiences this way:

> "... We talk about the dangers of vehicle extrication; I am clueless as to the internal workings of a car. Five months into the job, with all new gear that genuinely fits, and strength that is adequate for most situations, I am still perpetually handicapped by my ignorance of information that boys in our culture just seem to absorb." (p. 38)

Although it is not clear to me that boys absorb it more, they are clearly exposed to it more and that provides a bias that still exists.

A subcategory in the education and training concern was attitude. The women in the study commented that co-worker's attitude towards apprentices, in particular, female apprentices, affected the amount and kind of on-the-job training that was provided. Opportunities to learn through practice may be. withheld and, apprentices may not be provided with information on how to do work correctly and safely. In addition, sometimes incorrect health and safety practices are taught to apprentices. One woman said, ". . . when I came in and got some education and training, I thought 'whoop, I was lucky there I didn't get screwed up by getting injured on the job because I just flat really didn't know a lot about what was the correct way to do things.'" Another woman said, "and then there's a lot of people, . . . you know the younger ones that are coming up 'and they're out there and they're picking up these nasty crappy attitudes and stuff from the journeymen that they're working around because that's what they see 'em doing and it seems to work fine and you know, you can't combat that without an attitude change." This is again an area that closely parallels situations in fire and other emergency response fields.

According to some of the women, skill-based training did occur; however, it was done without the co-workers actually teaching. Most often it required the trainee to watch carefully to see the methods used by others. Although some women felt that it was a real benefit to watch the guys and pick up the tricks that make the job easier, other women felt that they were not being trained and they had to just figure things out for themselves. Additionally, the respondents said because they had less upper body strength, they had to be creative and develop ways to make the job possible and safe for a woman. As one woman said, ". . .I use my brain instead of my brawn."

Finally under education and training, supervisor influence was mentioned by many of the women, For example, one woman said, "Many (of the group) don't want to go to safety meetings. I don't know if it's a machismo thing or what, they're getting paid. But then there's always the contractor or boss breathing down your neck, saying, 'how come this wasn't done?' The boss doesn't say, 'you'd better go to that safety meeting because I don't want my worker's comp bill going up this year.' Contractors hate to see people sitting around."

The fourth area of safety concern was awareness of surroundings. The respondents felt that just knowing what was going on around them with regard to tools and equipment, being organized in their work and tools and in using good common sense is a safety issue. For example, one woman said, "You have to be aware of where your tools are, your surroundings. Very many times we've been in situations where we'd have to move very quickly or maybe be blind-sided and if we're not organized and know our surroundings, things can happen quick."

23

Although these women wanted others to be aware of health and safety issues on the job, they said they would not depend on others for their health and safety.

The final category of issues identified by these women had to do with health and safety issues associated with being a woman in the construction industry. The three issues of greatest concern in this category were lack of protective clothing and tools designed to fit a woman, feeling the need to overcompensate to prove oneself, and the lack of clean or, in many cases, any rest room facilities. These, I am sure, seem very familiar because they are directly paralleled in the fire and emergency response field.

Clearly having properly fitting clothing and equipment is a key health and safety issue. I hope that NIOSH will be able to take a lead in this area in terms of getting appropriately sized clothing for women, Although smaller women were affected to a greater degree by this issue, almost all of the women shared this concern. One woman said, "When I went through the welding apprenticeship . . . they issued us welding boots size 9-1/2. I had to wear 2 pair of socks to wear them. They gave me a welding leather jacket that was a foot longer than my hand, I had to roll it up. And they said that they couldn't order anything smaller. They gave me gloves, humongous; I couldn't even pick anything up." Another said, "They do not make hand tools for women and women come in all sizes, just like men. They need to get in touch with apprenticeship programs, with contractors, and push to have women's work boots and women's gloves for nontraditional trades. The information is not getting out there."

The second issue in this area is overcompensation. Women often said that they felt that they had to overcompensate to prove themselves to their co-workers and bosses. This bears out the statement from *A Handbook on Women in Firefighting* that,

> Members of a dominant group within any institution tend to view those who are not members of that group with skepticism. One way this dynamic affects women firefighters is in a strong insistence that they prove themselves by doing everything the hard way. (p. 9)

Here, again, we have a clear overlap in concerns. One woman construction worker said, "A lot of times, I feel like I've got to do this because I'm a girl because if I don't they're going to say, 'See, whad I tell ya. She's a girl, she can't lift it.' And I did, I ended up getting myself injured. It took once and one time only. I won't do it again, I won't be too proud to ask for help." At least one woman in the group found that her co-workers treated her like a little sister and offered help whenever they thought she needed it. She found this positive; however, she was often assigned less interesting tasks.

Finally,. the issue of available and clean bathroom facilities was discussed at length in these focus groups. Most participants said that if there were facilities available they were filthy. This again is an area of common concern with female firefighters. In *A Handbook on Women in Firefighting,* one observer wrote:

> Under the best circumstances, bad facilities are an inconvenience which women suffer from in far greater proportion. Under the worst conditions, poor facilities can lead to problems with morale and job performance, and an increase in the occurrence of harassment. . ." (p. 53; Linda Willing, "Bedrooms and Bathrooms: the Hidden Message," WFS *Quarterly,* Winter 1988-89, pp. 1-2)

Although this is a bit different with sleeping facilities in the fire station, there is a commonality of issues here. The inconvenience and harassment are there. A number of the women in construction mentioned that they will not go to the rest room until they can find a clean facility at lunchtime. I am looking for data to determine whether there is an increase risk for urinary tract infections and other health issues, as well as just an esthetics issue.

In terms of stress on the job, all of these issues are causes of stress. Most of these women did not talk about harassment unless probed.

Since construction is expected to be one of the few areas with future blue-collar employment potential, it is important to have a pool of men and women who have been both skill and safety trained and 'are ready to work. Apprenticeship and pre-apprenticeship programs should include realistic expectations of the job and how to exist within the dominant male culture. If women come to the jobsite without proper training, their presence at the worksite is less likely to be accepted, the view that women are hired only to meet quotas will be reinforced, and they may not get the on-the-job training which could result in high turnover or, worse yet, job-related injuries.

In 1979, an anthropologist named Jeffrey Reimer wrote that journeymen will have to adjust to having women enter the trades and that they may even benefit from them. He states that the integration of women may improve how work gets done and the quality of the finished product. While there has been some progress in integrating women into the construction workforce and into the emergency response force as well, we as safety and health professionals need to listen to the workers and continue to keep the doors open and make it a safe and healthy entry for women into these nontraditional fields.

RISK AND FEMALE FIRST RESPONDERS

Marko Bourne
Executive Director
Pennsylvania Fire Services Institute

I will be speaking today about risks faced by firefighters from an insurance perspective. We all have to deal with the insurance industry one way or another. The insurance industry has been very much involved with the fire service for a long time. Many of the companies that you know about, such as Volunteer Fireman's Insurance Services (VFIS) and the Provident and others, actually insure fire departments, firefighters, and emergency medical service organizations. In spite of their long history, they are just beginning to look at the risks confronted by firefighters, both men and women, and EMTs around the country. At this point they are just starting to gather the data needed to evaluate these risks.

The Centers for Disease Control (CDC), in their recently published book *Injury in America,* state that firefighting is one area where there is not enough statistical information gathered for them to draw any conclusions on how to change risk and behavior. The NFA, NFPA, and the USFA have been gathering data on firefighter death and injury for nearly twenty years, yet the information that the CDC needs is not available. It is very difficult to address risk and behavioral change issues if you do not have the numbers to support change. But some numbers do exist and let's look at them.

First, what is risk? Webster's dictionary defines risk as "a dangerous element or factor, the chance of loss." Insurance companies use a slightly different definition, "The chance of loss or peril to a subject, the degree of probability of loss or anything that it specifies and a hazard to an insurer." As you can see, if you think about it, that could be absolutely anything. Particularly anything we do in fire/response professions.

Workers' compensation and disability rates are based on the insurance industry's understanding of what the risks are. That is one of the reasons workers' compensation reform is a big issue in Pennsylvania, because no one knew just what the risks are. As firefighters and EMTs, we are in an inherently risky profession, more so than most others, and this has been borne out by statistics over the years.

The following are some statistics from Pennsylvania between 1990 and 1992. In that time period, firefighter deaths in Pennsylvania totaled twenty-seven. Over 50 percent of them were heart related. This is a major risk factor. Most of those who died of heart attack were between the ages of 44 and 66. This is a common age range for heart related deaths across the nation, What I was interested in was what they were doing when they had their attacks. One was operating the pump, which is not really a stressful situation, usually. One was responding to a fire, one responding to an automatic alarm, one directing traffic, two were operating hoseline in fire situations, and one was a training session death. Only the two who were operating in a fire were in what we would normally consider high risk. But a lot goes back to physical fitness

26

and personal behaviors, which need to be addressed as well. Of the deaths in the period we are discussing, 4 percent were females, and that matches the percentage of females in the fire department. There seems to be no less risk for female firefighters to have fireground death or injury than any other firefighters.

Other deaths in the same period in Pennsylvania had to do with collapsed structures, vehicle accidents, and lost in a structure. The one that stands out as a problem is a training incident-and training is an area where death or injury is hardest to absolve. These sessions should be designed for trainees to learn but not get hurt. A recent national study indicated that women stand an equal probability of heart problems as men. In the last four years, there has only been one heart attack related claim for a woman to one of the insurance companies. It came from Florida and occurred in a training environment. It was a simulated smoke environment in a house-a 26-year-old woman crawling into the house collapsed, never regained consciousness, and died. The report states that she was a volunteer white female and she died of a cardiac arrhythmia (a complication of a hereditary condition). Could this have been prevented? Possibly. There are certain kinds of testing that can identify these pre-existing problems so they can be dealt with through behavioral change. I use this case as an illustration that women are facing heart problem in the fire service as well as in the national study group mentioned above.

The VFIS has provided data on claims from 1990-94. Of 135 death claims received, 6 were women, This represents 4 percent of the total claims, which is close to the ratio of women currently in career or volunteer fire service. Injury statistics seem to follow about the same pattern. It is incumbent on us to begin to identify ways to reduce risk. Insurance providers use loss control, whereby they send experts to sites to identify site and process hazards and advise companies of what to do to reduce their chance of loss. Loss control for the fire service is what we do to prevent the loss of lives as well. Risk control is actually a form of loss control for people.

According to *Injury in America,* there are three approaches to loss control:

1. **Persuasion.** Getting people to recognize behaviors and practices that need to be altered and alter them. Examples of persuasion include getting people to install and use smoke detectors or to stop smoking by using informational or advertising campaigns. In fire school, we often train people by rote and train not to do specific things on the fire ground.

2. **Requirement.** This method relies on a law or standard operating procedure (SOP) to force change of behavior or practices that need to be altered. Examples of this level of risk control include a SOP that requires the use of gloves and masks on EMS calls and seat belt laws.

3. **Automatic Protection.** This is building inherent safeguards into the things we use and our environment to keep us safe. Examples of this type of risk control are sprinkler systems and air bags.

We must be careful, though, because you cannot depend on any one of the approaches alone. Any one of the methods can only go so far because the "human element" often leads to individuals to get around requirements and automatic systems.

Work has been going on in risk control in industry. There are reams of information on all kinds of industries, but very little that relates to firefighting. The National Research Council made several recommendations on ways to improve risk management. First, education and training programs must be evaluated experimentally to determine whether they are working and what they actually do to improve or change behavior. Second, product design research must be constantly examined or reexamined to expedite provision of more automatic safety measures. With this, it is essential to acknowledge the human factors that will come into play. Finally, research into the "people barriers" is needed. Exactly what are the factors that encourage or discourage people from doing what they know will reduce the risks they face?

The program here this weekend is important because it will identify issues that need to be addressed for both women and men firefighters and first responders. We need to keep a balance between our individuality and the need to teach people coming into the system how they should operate in a safe manner. It is critical that we avoid knee-jerk reactions to change that will reduce or eliminate behavioral change. In conclusion, we must examine life safety in the fire and emergency services in the same way that they do in industry. The losses that we incur far outweigh our numbers. Therefore, we must undertake a serious examination of our operation with an eye to our own loss control and reduce our injuries and deaths before someone else does it for us.

ADDRESSING HEALTH AND INJURY ISSUES: ANTICIPATING AND PREPARING

Jeff Dyar
EMS Chairperson, National Fire Academy

Historically, the emergency response organization has taken a post-active or crisis management approach to safety. When something occurs, such as an obvious safety violation, we act on it. This mode of operation is also known, more technically, as the catastrophic theory of reform.

Now spurred on by anticipatory acts, such as rules, regulations, laws or standards from insurance companies, we are changing how we will operate. We are trying to change to a proactive approach. A text, *Injury in America, a Continuing Public Health Problem* published in 1985 and updated in 1989 by the Committee on Trauma Research, Commission on Life Sciences, National Research Council, and the Institute of Medicine, suggested specific ways to deal with injury prevention and safety. Have we made any inroads on the trends and have we listened to what they recommended? They recommended a three-phase approach to dealing with injury prevention from a training and awareness standpoint:

1. Persuade-alter behavior to a self protection mode
2. Require-apply a law or administrative rule
3. Provide automatic protection-product or environmental design

These steps are characteristic of how an organization solves safety problems in terms of how we have been training people. For example, if a study says we are not using our seat belts, the chief will get up and say, "Now, we really ought to be wearing our belts whenever we go out, " and there may be a nice memo to the effect that we must wear our belts. That is the course that will draw the least resistance, so it is a relatively comfortable place to be organizationally. Then the chief sees the fire truck drive by with a crew that is not using the belts, so a rule that says "thou shalt be belted or thou will lose a days pay" is made. That gets people's attention and you begin to get some compliance. Finally, the chief goes to a conference where the chiefs get together and draft a standard with some guidelines. Often the next step is a federal regulation or law which has teeth and can cost the jurisdiction money. Finally, someone decides that the best solution is to automate the belts so whenever someone sits in the seat the belt will close and no one has to push or persuade anyone.

In terms of effectiveness, these methods usually proceed in reverse order, with persuasion lowest. There are some cases where laws and regulations have worked such as helmet laws. This is also very visible; it is impossible to ride a bike down the street without everyone knowing whether the driver is wearing a helmet; therefore, it is more enforceable. Automatic protection is often more effective because people do not have to think about it to do it. It might be better to start with the third approach and get on with being safer by building a safe environment. However, a combination of the methods may be the best solution.

The fire service does not have a research database to know what we are doing and not doing. In fact, in terms of gender issues, we do not keep gender-specific statistics. There are many kinds of data the fire service needs to collect. In fact, ten years ago the group said we needed to collect data and get a base point to supply some focus to our research and make it possible to share information. As far as I can see, we have not made much progress in that area in the last ten years.

High risk groups tend to be harder to sell in terms of behavioral changes. The personality traits or characteristics of emergency responders have been described as action-oriented risk takers, even to the point of being obsessive compulsive in many cases. These are aggressive over-achievers who are not necessarily good at sorting out safe behaviors through a decision-making process. In the fire service, we want people who will run toward the fire, but recognize that there are responsibilities with that.

Meanwhile, we have to use a modified stick-and-carrot approach. In South Carolina they have mandated that NFPA 1582 be adopted by all departments. This happened because the number and cost of injury claims had become a problem and they had to do something about it. The unacceptable risk is driving insurance companies which are driving the implementation of safety measures.

At the National Fire Academy (NFA) we have built curriculum for safety. About seven years ago we started with *Safety and Survival: the Company Officer's Role,* which had to do with providing company officers with some alternatives in terms of safety. We were in a persuasion mode at that time. The second course at that time was *Health and Safety Program Implementation.* This course was a guideline on how to build a program within your department. This, too, was in persuasion mode because it had no means of requiring implementation. Just about two weeks ago, a new pair of courses, *Incident Safety Officer* and *Health and Safety Officer,* were finished. They will be distributed through state services training organizations.

These courses were built to meet needs identified by experts across the country. We added a section on risk management and discovered that there is a fundamental deficiency in understanding what risk is and what risk is acceptable and unacceptable. Risk management is divided into three categories:

Training Activities. Injury in this category is unacceptable because this is a predictable and controllable environment and if it is controlled correctly injury can be avoided.

Pre-emergency. This is proactive risk management in which we identify possible problems and evaluate frequency and severity to determine any connection and prioritize actions to take to avoid risk.

Emergency Settings. Incident safety officer goes to these settings. This position is mandated at hazardous materials incidents and should be at all operational scenes.

When these courses were developed, we tried to use the three-phase approach to safety:

- Identify issues and encourage changes in behavior,
- Mandate changes through rules and regulations, then
- Build things safer to eliminate or reduce risks.

This is the direction that the Academy is taking with regard to safety. We will now take it to the response community, encouraging them to combine these steps with agencywide efforts to anticipate and prepare for safe operation.

30

FEMALE FIRST RESPONDER HEALTH AND SAFETY: ENHANCING RESOURCES THAT PROTECT THE COMMUNITY

Lynn Oliver, Deputy Chief
Kirkland Fire Department

In July 1983, I was introduced to the City Council in Mercer Island, Washington, as the new Fire Chief. I knew it was a really big step to move from fire prevention to chief in a small community, but what really got my attention and made me realize the position I had gotten myself into was what happened a few days later. I was in my office when one of the guys came into my office and said, "Chief, there is a reporter from CNN who wants to interview you." As I stood in the apparatus bay and answered the questions of this reporter, I could feel the responsibility and weight of what I had taken on coming around me. What I realized was how important it was for me to do well to do right because I was representing all women. I was convinced that, if I made a mistake, it would not be a fire chief making an inappropriate decision, it would be, "Look they hired a woman and look how she did."

As you can imagine, I set out really working hard .to do that good job working collaboratively with the people in my department and my region. It was really important to me to gain the respect of my peer professionals, the other Fire Chiefs in my region and my state, so I got really myopic about that. What happened then was that I got out of touch with what was happening with women in the rest of the fire service. When I occasionally checked in I saw that the numbers in my region were growing and that Women in the Fire Service (WFS) was organized to network and nurture women on the national level. So I had the idea that things are moving along and we are doing OK.

Then I was invited to do a series of programs in Orlando, instructing women firefighters who came from all over the US, but primarily the eastern part of the country. We were covering women's issues, wanting to provide empowerment, solutions to problems, and so on. It started slowly, but the stories came out. The one mentioned here the other day about the glass in the bunker boots is a true story.

Just to give you an idea, here are a few situations that came out of these classes. What would you do if:

You were patted on the butt by the chief of the department? Where would you go?

Crew members spit in your coffee?

Your battalion chief completed your performance evaluation with a kiss?

You were videotaped taking a shower and learned later that the video tape had been shared with all the members of your department?

These were just some samples of the situations that came out in the classes, and I bring them out today to reinforce that it is important to be sure that we do not get stuck in our own track and forget that these things are still going on. In our group, several examples came out of calls

31

in the last few days about people who are still not getting equitable treatment within their departments. Even though we are working really hard, it is important to continue to support one another.

Last year, the department where I work now hired its first female firefighter. What I learned then was that it is like 1974 all over again. All the same old questions were coming up. There may be transference of what we learn at the intellectual level, but certainly not at the gut level. The message to me was that each time a fire department hires its first female or promotes its first female Lieutenant, Battalion Chief, Chief, whatever, it is **breaking new ground.** Each fire department must painfully experience all of the problems and issues itself. There is little transference at this time.

I am encouraged that more departments are hiring their first female and promoting their first female. We all just sat here and clapped when it was announced that another department had hired a chief of a department who is a woman. I would submit to you that the true achievement will be when it is not significant at all that a woman was hired into this position.

We have had two days to reflect on issues that preserve the health and safety of women in roles of first responders and those who are yet to join us. It is very clear that these women have a vital role in the well being of our communities. We have drafted the outline of action steps to be taken at the federal, state, and local levels. I would divide the steps we have defined into two categories. First, the concrete measures, such as developing clear policies, having bunker gear that fits, improving our administrative practices from hiring throughout the period of employment, and undertaking research specific to the reproductive health and toxicological issues faced by women first responders. Second, the more subtle, because we are looking at trying to find ways to actually make attitudinal changes and training managers to actually look for clues and ways to. support the mental health of their female employees as well as all their employees. We also are looking for ways to see women illustrated in informational and promotional media. I know that I really feel good when I see a Battalion Chief like Molly Douce being interviewed at an incident scene and there is no question woman or not that she is in charge.

I think we should feel really good about what we have done in the past couple of days. We have written prescriptions that will enhance the work of the female first responders by focusing on their health and safety. Now we can hand off to the U.S. Fire Administration with very high expectations. Women first responders around the country would be cheering if they knew what we were doing. I'd like to thank Carrye Brown, Administrator, U. S. Fire Administration, for her support.

I am looking forward to hearing the word **"firefighter"** without the word female in front of it. We will be referring to .all the members on the force.

CLOSING REMARKS

Carrye B. Brown, Administrator
U.S. Fire Administration

Thank you for coming to this important event. The firefighter community is changing. The number of women, while still a low percentage, is increasing rapidly. For example, last week the first female fire chief was appointed in Prince William County, Virginia. What was significant according to press accounts was that she was selected to run a department with problems in morale, staffing, and the use of resources. The philosophy of selecting the best person for the job is now found throughout America and that is very encouraging. It is more important now than ever before that we have this and other symposiums to address the health and safety needs of female firefighters and other first responders and that's why I'm here because if the position that I'm in can lend any weight to the importance of it I want to be here to say that. To say that to my staff, to FEMA, and to the community at large. These are issues that we have to take seriously and look at together.

Looking over the schedule of the symposium, I can see what a valuable conference this has been. Thank you for giving your weekend to this effort. Thank you to Jean Adams who has worked so hard to ensure the success of this symposium. By being here, I want to express and demonstrate to you the importance that I feel for the issues you have been talking about and that there will be follow-up to this. I have a very outstanding staffer who will keep me on track on these issues.

Finally, as the Administrator of the USFA, we are committed to address the needs of our customers-the fire service community. I want us to always work toward improving fire safety for both women and men. This conference will help as we receive your input and plan for future activities. There is strength in our numbers and there is strength in our working together collectively.

TASK FORCE SYMPOSIUM

HEALTH AND SAFETY ISSUES
OF
THE FEMALE EMERGENCY RESPONDER

WESTPARK HOTEL
ARLINGTON, VIRGINIA

OCTOBER 29-31, 1994

SYMPOSIUM GOALS

¤ To identify and define key issues related to the health and
safety of female firefighters and first responders

¤ To develop strategies that address health and injury related
concerns for female firefighters and first responders

¤ To prioritize actions that can be used to implement strategies
confronting health and injury considerations of female
firefighters and first responders

Agenda

8:30 a.m.

Registration
The Dogwood Room

9:00 a.m.

Welcoming Remarks
  Jean Adams
  Project Officer
  Fire Technical Programs
  U.S. Fire Administration

9:10 a.m.

Introductions and Overview
  Kenneth H. Stewart
  Stewart Training Associates

9:30 a.m.

"Tradeswomen's Perspectives on Occupation Health and Safety"
  Linda M. Goldenbar, Ph.D.
  Division of Surveillance, Hazard Evaluations and
    Field Studies
  National Institute for Occupational Health
    and Safety

10:00 a.m.

Break

10:20 a.m.

Focus Group Research
Issues in Female First Responder Health and Safety

- Procedures, Protocols, and Equipment
- Organizational and Mental Health
- Reproductive and Toxicological

  Kenneth H. Stewart

12:00 p.m.

LUNCH, THE GEORGETOWN ROOM

"Risk and Female First Responders"
  Marko Bourne
  Executive Director
  Pennsylvania Fire Services Institute

Afternoon Session

1:15 p.m.   Focus Group Research, The Dogwood Room
                                   Kenneth H. Stewart

2:30 p.m.   Break

2:45 p.m.   Focus Group Research Presentations and Discussion
                                   Kenneth H. Stewart

6:30 p.m.   **DINNER**

Sunday, October 30, 1994
Morning Session

10:00 a.m.   Welcome, The Dogwood Room

                                   "Addressing Health and Injury Issues: Anticipating and
                                   Preparing"
                                   Jeff Dyar
                                   EMS Chairperson
                                   National Fire Academy

10:30 a.m.   Focus Group Discussions

12:00 p.m.   **LUNCH, THE GEORGETOWN ROOM**

Afternoon Session

1:15 p.m.   Focus Group Discussions, The Dogwood Room
                                   Kenneth H. Stewart

2:15 p.m.   Break

2:30 p.m.   Focus Group Presentations
                                   "Strategies to Address Female First Responder
                                   Health and Safety Issues"
                                   Kenneth H. Stewart

6:30 p.m.   **DINNER**

8:00 a.m.   Focus Group Discussions, The Dogwood Room
                             Kenneth II. Stewart

9:00 a.m.   Focus Group Presentations
                             "Priority Actions and Responsibilities to
                             Address Female First Responder Health and
                             Safety Issues"
                             Kenneth H. Stewart

10:00 a.m.   Break

10:15 a.m.   "Female First Responder Health and Safety:
                             Enhancing Resources that Protect the
                             Community"
                             Lynn Oliver, Deputy Chief
                             Kirkland Fire Department

10:35 a.m.   Closing Remarks
                             Carrye B. Brown
                             Administrator
                             U.S. Fire Administration

10:40 a.m.   Focus Group Research
                             Issues in Female First Responder Health and Safety

                             ■ Procedures, Protocols, and Equipment
                             ■ Organizational and Mental Health
                             ■ Reproductive and Toxicological

                             Kenneth H. Stewart

Health and Safety Issues of the Female Emergency Responder

Westpark Hotel
Arlington, Virginia

October 29-31, 1994

Speakers and Participants

Dee S. Armstrong
President
Women in the Fire Service
Fairfax County Fire Department
Fairfax, VA 22030

Sharon Doyle Arndt
Safety and Health Assistant
Department of Occupational Health & Safety
International Association of Fire Fighters
Washington, D.C. 20006

Karen M. Barber
Paramedic
Orange County Fire & Rescue Department
Orlando, FL 32807

Marko Bourne
Executive Director
Pennsylvania Fire Services Institute
Harrisburg, PA 17101

Diane P. Breedlove
Chief
Sugar Land Fire Department
Sugar Land, TX 77478

Betty Brown
Lieutenant
Hampton Fire Department, Station 10
Hampton, VA 23666

Carrye B. Brown
Administrator
United States Fire Administration
Federal Emergency Management Agency
Emmitsburg, MD 21727

Kenneth Brown
Senior Engineer
ARCCA, Inc.
Richboro, PA 18954

Paul D. Brown
Instructor
Maryland Fire and Rescue Institute
University of Maryland
College Park, MD 20742

Molly Ann Douce
Battalion Chief
Seattle Fire Department
Seattle, WA 98117

Jeff Dyar
EMS Chairman
National Fire Academy
Emmitsburg, MD 21727

Pat A. Dyas
Captain
Shreveport Fire Department
Shreveport, LA 71101

Jim Fisher
Emergency Medical Technician
Hampton Township EMS
Mechanicsburg, PA 17055

Stephanie Fisher
Emergency Medical Technician
Pennsylvania Emergency Health
    Services Council
Mechanicsburg, PA 17055

Stephen N. Foley
Senior Fire Services Safety Specialist
National Fire Protection Association
Quincy, MA 02169

Linda M. Goldenhar, Ph.D.
Health Behavior Researcher
National Institute for Occupational
    Safety & Health
Cincinnati, OH 45226-1998

Mark S. Lawler
Chairman
Aircraft Rescue Fire Fighting
    Working Group
Honolulu, HI 96820

Eileen Lewis
Assistant Chief of Administration
Tacoma Fire Department
Tacoma, MD 98402

Mark Nugent
Senior Captain
Chesterfield Fire Department
Chesterfield, VA 23832

Lynn Oliver
Deputy Chief
Kirkland Fire Department
Kirkland, WA 98035

Francine Ourada
Captain
Hampton Fire Department
Hampton, VA 23669

Billy Rutherford
Human Factors Engineer
JFR, Inc.
Springfield, VA 22153

Jim Schamadan, MD
Medical Director
Phoenix Fire Department
Scottsdale, AZ 85251

Denise Stein
Clinical Nurse Specialist
Franklin Square Hospital
Baltimore, MD 21237

Scott Stein
Project Manager
York Hospital Foundation
York, PA 17405

Julie Wheeler
Occupational Health and Safety Director
Hazardous Waste Coordinator
Rogue River National
Medford, OR 97501

HEALTH AND SAFETY NEEDS OF
THE FEMALE EMERGENCY RESPONDER

SUGGESTED READING

PRE-CONFERENCE

Elo, Anna-Liisa. 1994. Assessment of mental stress factors at work. In *Occupational Medicine*. 3rd ed. Edited by Carl Zenz, O. Bruce Dickerson, and Edward P. Horvath, Jr. St. Louis: Mosby-Year Book, Inc. Ch. 57:945-59.

Federal Emergency Management Agency/U. S . Fire Administration. 1993. *The changing face of the fire service: A handbook on women in firefighting.* FA- 128.

Poitrast, Bruce J., and Carl Zenz. 1994. Women in the workplace: Introductory considerations. In *Occupational Medicine*. 3rd ed. Edited by Carl Zenz, 0. Bruce, and Edward P. Horvath, Jr. St. Louis: Mosby-Year Book, Inc., Ch. 57:827-35.

Scott, Allene J., and Joseph LaDou. 1994. Health and safety in shift workers. In *Occupational Medicine*. 3rd ed. Edited by Carl Zenz, O. Bruce Dickerson, and Edward P. Horvath, Jr. St. Louis: Mosby-Year Book, Inc. Ch. 67:960-86.

ISSUE 1 - PROCEDURES, PROTOCOLS, AND EQUIPMENT ISSUES

PERSONAL PROTECTIVE EQUIPMENT

Bone, Jan. 1992. PPE gives workers a fighting chance. *Safety & Health* (September): 34-36.

Coletta, Gerard C., Irving J. Arons, Louis E. Ashley, and Arthur P. Drerman. 1976. *The development of criteria for firefighters' gloves. Vol. 2, Glove criteria and test methods.* Washington, D.C. DHEW (NIOSH) Publication No. 77-134-B, February 1976.

Federal Emergency Management Agency, U. S . Fire Administration. 1980. FA-7, *Model performance criteria for structural firefighters' helmets.* FA-7. August 1977.

Federal Emergency Management Agency, U. S . Fire Administration. 1993. *Protective clothing and equipment needs of emergency responders for urban search and rescue missions.*

Gauen, Pat. 1993. Firefighters see light at tunnel's end. *St. Louis Post Dispatch (SL)* (17 May 1993):1.

Hillsgrove, Sandy. 1989-90. Someone is finally listening. WFS Quarterly (winter): 13-14.

Kelley, Martin. C. 1978. Turnouts for safety. *Firehouse* (April):45, 60.

Larussa, Robert. 1987. More safety in protective clothing sought by industry, government. *Daily News Record (22* September 1987):S2-3.

Lawrence, J. Richard. 1987. Protective clothing: A new materials update. *Fire Command* (September):48-49.

McNamee, James J. 1984. Safety comes first in Cleveland. *Fire Engineering* (November): 40-42.

Minter, Stephen G. 1989. ISEA focuses on the future. *Occupational Hazards* (July):9(3).

National Institute for Occupational Safety and Health. 1987. NIOSH respirator decision logic. Subcommittee of the NIOSH Respiratory Protection Committee. DHHS (NIOSH) Publication No. 87-108. NIOSH, Centers for Disease Control, PHS, USDHHS.

Reischl, Uwe. 1986, Fire fighter helmet ventilation analysis. *Am. Ind. Hyg. Assoc. J.* 47, no. 8:546-551.

Russell, David. 1983. Seven fire fighters caught in explosion. *Fire Engineering* (April): 22-23.

Stormen, Steve, and James H. Veghte. 1991. *Qualitatively evaluating the comfort, fit, function and integrity of chemical protective suit ensembles,* FEMA/USFA, FA- 107, 1991. Final Report, Task 2.

Veghte, James H. 1983. Protective clothing survey results. *Fire Service Today* (August): 16-19.

White, Mary Kay, and Thomas K. Hodous. 1988. Physiological responses to the wearing of fire fighter's turnout gear with neoprene and GORE-TEX" barrier liners. *Am. Ind. Hyg. Assoc. J.* 49 (October):523-30.

TRAINING AND TESTING

Bird, James W. 1991. Training women for the P.A.T. *Fire Engineering* (March):87-93.

Crimmins, Jerry. 1994. So many jobs, so little time: Firefighters dousing image of old job. *Chicago Tribune.* 10 February 1994. Metro section: 1.

Federal Emergency Management Agency, U. S , Fire Administration. 1990. FA-95. *Physical fitness coordinator's manual for fire departments.*

Floren, Terese M. 1991, 1992. A study in litigation. *WFS Quarterly.* Part 1 (fall):12-13; Part 2 (winter): 10-12.

George, Arthur E. 1988. Only one standard. *Fire Engineering* (March):37-38.

Hirschman, Jessica. 1993. Climbing the glass ladder, part 1. *Firefighter's News.* (April/May) : 62-67

Hirschman, Jessica. 1993. Climbing the glass ladder, part 2. *Firefighter's News.* (July):44-47.

Lovvorn, Allan W., Douglas Voltolina, Louis R. Bainbridge, Larry B. Anderson, M. Ray Brown, and Edward W. White. 1990. Women in fire suppression, where are they? Applied research project submitted to the National Fire Academy as part of the Executive Fire Officer Program. 15-26 January 1990.

Wasylyk, Sylvia. 1994. Women in the fire service: Issues and answers. *The Voice* (September):38-41.

Women's training program upgrades firefighting skills. 1991. *Fire Chief* (February): 60-61.

Women's training program in Jacksonville. 1991. *WFS Quarterly 6(2):* 1-3.

ISSUE 2 - O RGANIZATIONAL & M ENTAL HEALTH ISSUES

ACCEPTANCE

Balazs, Diana. 1993. Burning barriers: Woman firefighter breaks ground with promotion to captain. *Arizona Republic/Phoenix Gazette,* Northwest Community, (23 August 1993):1.

City of Seattle Fire Department. n.d. Women in the Seattle Fire Department: Results of questionaire and interviews.

Cohn, D'Vera, and Barbara Vobejda. 1992. For women, uneven strides in workplace. *The Washington Post.* 21 December 1992, A: 1.

Ecenbarger, William. 1984. Are volunteer fire companies coming to the end of their ladder? *Philadelphia Inquirer Magazine* (7 October 1984): 16.

Hallinan, Lorin. 1994. Breaking the barriers. *Emergency* (May):32-37.

Kaufman, Leslie. 1994. Women come aboard. *Government Executive.* (July):40-43.

Keagan, Anne. 1991. Hot Seat. *Chicago Tribune Magazine.* 8 September 1991. 14, 16, 18, 20, 32.

Kurh, Mary Chris. 1987. Some women face battle to fight fires. *Times Union* (Albany NY), 12 October 1987, B-1.

McGraw, Erin. 1987. Women at work: Firefighting hooks her a first for Manchester. *Boston Globe* (18 October 1987), New Hampshire Week.

McQueen, Iris. 1990. Blowing smoke. *The California Fire Service* (September):12-15, 21.

---1990. Females in fire operations: Nightmare or dreamscape for the 90's. *The California Fire Service* (April): 14-15, 17.

McRoberts, Flynn, 1993. Women blaze new trails in firefighting. *Chicago Tribune (26 March 1993)* DU: 1.

Miller, Kathy, Ellen Rosell, and Karen Barber. n.d. Fighting fires and sexual harassment.

Pankowski, Karen. 1992. Firefighter wants her suspension reviewed. *Orlando Sentinel (29 May 1992)* B:3.

Peart, Karen N. Women at work. *Scholastic Update* 125 (12 March 1993):8(4).

Poitrast, Bruce J., and Carl Zenz. 1994. Women in the workplace: Introductory considerations. In *Occupational Medicine.* 3rd ed. Edited by Carl Zenz, 0. Bruce, and Edward P. Horvath, Jr. St. Louis: Mosby-Year Book, Inc., Ch. 57:827-35.

Sturzenacker, Gloria. 1986. Prejudice prevention. *Chief Fire Executive* (April-May) 1986:43-45, 76, 78.

Warshaw, Robin. 1994. Getting into smoke-filled rooms. *Philadelphia Inquirer Magazine* (11 September 1994):20-24, 28.

Yaskin, Joseph. 1994. When things get hot, this fire official knows how to hold her own. *Philadelphia Inquirer,* (30 January 1994):G-6.

STRESS

Behling, Debra, and Judi Guy. 1993. Hazards of the healthcare profession. *Occupational Health & Safety* 62, no. 2 (February):54-57.

Bruening, John C. 1988. Women's stress quotient is climbing. *Occupational Hazards* (August):45-47.

Elo, Anna-Liisa. 1994. Assessment of mental stress factors at work. In *Occupational Medicine.* 3rd ed. Edited by Carl Zenz, O. Bruce Dickerson, and Edward P. Horvath, Jr. St. Louis: Mosby-Year Book, Inc. Chap. 57:945-59.

Federal Emergency Management Agency/U. S. Fire Administration. 1991, Stress management: Model program for maintaining firefighter well-being. FA-100.

Glazner, Linda K. 1992. Shift work and its effects on fire fighters and nurses. *Occupational Health & Safety* 6 (July):43-46.

James, Alma E.C., and Peter L. Wright. 1993. Perceived locus of control: Occupational stress in the ambulance service. *Journal of Managerial Psychology 8:3-8.*

Scott, Allene J., and Joseph LaDou. 1994. Health and safety in shift workers. In *Occupational Medicine.* 3rd ed. Edited by Carl Zenz, O. Bruce Dickerson, and Edward P. Horvath, Jr. St. Louis: Mosby-Year Book, Inc. Ch. 67:960-86.

Spenser, Steven. 1993. A paramedic's life: Street grit, saving lives, job can be difficult and stressful, but it has its rewards. *Seattle Times,* September 12, 1993. Business Section, p. J-1.

Spicer, John. 1988. Workplace stress worse for women. *Times of London,* July 4, 1988, Labour Research Department Report,

Stilwell, J.A., and P. J. Stilwell. 1984. Sickness absence in an ambulance service. *J. Soc. Occup. Med.* (England) 34/3:96-99.

Wooton, Jan P. 1991. The national sleep deficit: Are we snoozing into disaster? *Professional Safety* 36, no. 8:14-21.

ISSUE 3 - REPRODUCTIVE AND TOXICOLOGICAL ISSUES

CANCER

International Association of Fire Fighters. 1982. *Occupational Cancer and the Fire Fighter.*

HEARING LOSS

Freedman, Alan J. 1993. Hearing loss: An avoidable hazard. *Fire Engineering* (April):69-70, 72-75.

Niland, Jill, and Carl Zenz. 1994. Occupational hearing loss, noise, and hearing conservation. In *Occupational Medicine.* 3rd ed. Edited by Carl Zenz, O. Bruce Dickerson, and Edward P. Horvath, Jr. St. Louis: Mosby-Year Book, Inc. Chap.21:258-96.

Suter, Alice H., and John R. Franks, eds. 1990. A practical guide to effective hearing conservation programs in the workplace. NIOSH Publication No. 90-120.

HEART DISEASE

Bates, John Terence. 1987. Coronary artery disease deaths in the Toronto fire department. *Journal of Occupational Medicine* 29, no. 2 (February): 132-35.

Bledsoe, Bryan E., and Dwayne E. Clayden. 1993. Recognizing and managing angina pectoris. *JEMS* (August): 22-25, 79-83, 86-87.

Dibbs, Elaine, H. Emerson Thomas, Jr., Scott T. Weiss, and David Sparrow. 1982. Fire fighting and coronary heart disease. *Circulation* 65 (5):943-45.

Ferguson, Earl W. n.d. Detection of coronary artery disease in fire fighters without symptoms: Routine exercise testing is inadequate.

Fisher, Jeffrey D. The firefighter's guide to cardiovascular disease. 1992. *Firehouse* (August):42-49.

Handberg, Eileen, and Todd Keith. 1992. Clot busters: The future of EMS thrombolytics. *JEMS* (April):74-75, 77-80, 83,

Kuorinka, Ilkka, and Olli Korhonen. 1981. Firefighters' reaction to alarm, an ECG and heart rate study. *Journal of Occupational Medicine* 23 (11) : 762-66.

Sardinas, Anthony, Julia Wang Miller, and Holger Hansen. 1986. Ischemic heart disease mortality of firemen and policemen. *American Journal of Public Health 76 (9):* 1140-41.

HEAT

Alabama University Medical Center. 1976. *Assessment of Deep Body Temperatures of Workers in Hot Jobs.* Birmingham AL: NIOSH Research Report, PB-274 705.

--- 1977. *Assessment of Deep Body Temperatures o   f Women in Hot Jobs.*   Birmingham AL: NIOSH Research Report, PB-274 769.

Arata, Michael J., Jr. 1993. Heat protection. *Occupational Health & Safety,* 50-51.

Donelan, Steve. 1994. How to treat the victim-and protect yourself. *Rescue* (July/August): 24-31.

Dorsey, Stephen M. 1993. Firefighting in hot weather: Surviving the heat stress factor. *Firehouse* (June) 30, 32, 96.

International Association of Fire Chiefs. 1991. Heat, noise, physical exertion may cause reproductive hazards for fire fighters. *Newsbriefs.*

Payne, W. R., B. Portier, I. Fairweather, S. Zhou, and R. Snow. 1994. Thermoregulatory response to wearing encapsulated protective clothing during simulated work in various thermal environments. *American Industrial Hygiene Association Jo urnal* 55 (6):529-36.

LUNG/RESPIRATORY

Cook, Chuck, and Maria Cone. 1963. Deadly smoke. *The Register* (December).

Forgue, Joseh M. Respiratory protection for fire fighters. 1992. *American Society of Safety Engineers* (November) : 37-40.

Garnham. 1994. TB or not TB. *Emergency* (June):45-49.

Kern, David C., Marguerite A. Neill, David S. Wrenn, and J. Curtis Varone. 1993. Investigation of a unique time-space cluster of sarcoidosis in firefighters, *American Review of Respiratory Disease*   148:974-80.

Musk, William, John M. Peters, and David H. Wegman. 1977. Lung function in fire fighters, I: A three year follow-up of active subjects. *American Journal of Public Health* 67: 626-29.

Sheppard, D., S. Distefano, L. Morse, and C. Becker. 1986. Acute effects of routine firefighting on lung function. *American Journal of Industrial Medicine* 9:333-40.

Sparrow, David, Raymond Bosse, Bernard Rosner, and Scott T. Weiss, 1982. The effect of occupational exposure on pulmonary function. *American Review of Respiratory Diseases* 125:319-22.

Viadana, Enrico, and Irwin D. J. Bross, and Lorne Houten. 1976. Cancer experience of men exposed to inhalation of chemicals or to combustion products. *Journal of Occupational Medicine* 18 (12):787-92.

REPRODUCTIVE

Castelli, Jim. 1992. Federal agencies encouraged to increase reproductive-hazard protection, *Safety & Health* (February):41-44.

Evanoff, Bradley A., and Linda Rosenstock. 1986. Reproductive hazards in the workplace: A case study of women firefighters. *American Journal of Industrial Medicine* 9:503-15.

Floren, Terese M. 1993. Health problems raise questions for NYC EMT's. *Women in the Fire Service.* 11 (6).

Reproductive toxicology and occupational exposure. 1994. In *Occupational Medicine.* 3rd. ed. Edited by Carl Zenz. O. Bruce, and Edward P. Horvath, Jr. St. Louis: Mosby-Year Book, Inc. Ch. 58:836-69.

www.ingramcontent.com/pod-product-compliance
Lightning Source LLC
Chambersburg PA
CBHW081229170526
45165CB00009B/3015